UNDERSTANDING DISEASE

The
COMMON COLD
and
INFLUENZA

UNDERSTANDING DISEASE

ARTHRITIS
THE COMMON COLD AND INFLUENZA
HEART DISEASE

UNDERSTANDING DISEASE

The
COMMON COLD
and
INFLUENZA

NANCY STEDMAN

Illustrated by Michael Reingold

Medical Consultant: Sarmistha Hauger, M.D.
Pediatric Department, Babies Hospital
Columbia-Presbyterian Medical Center, New York City

JULIAN MESSNER NEW YORK

Photos pp. 23 and 25 courtesy of the Centers for Disease Control, Atlanta, Ga.

Photo p. 41 courtesy of Dr. Steven Mostow, Rose Medical Center, Denver, Colo.

Color photos of rhino virus model and map courtesy of Dr. Michael G. Rossman, Purdue University, West Lafayette, Ind.

Manufactured in the United States of America

10 9 8 7 6 5 4 3 2

Library of Congress Cataloging in Publication Data

Stedman, Nancy.
  The common cold and influenza.

  (Understanding disease)
  Includes index.
  Summary: Describes colds and influenza, the nature of the viruses that cause them, how they spread, methods of prevention and treatment, and the research for future cures.
    1. Influenza – Juvenile literature.   2. Cold (Disease) – Juvenile literature.
  [1. Influenza.   2. Cold Disease)]   I. Title.   II. Series.   [DNLM: 1. Common Cold – popular works.   2. Influenza – popular works.   WC 510 S812c]
  RC150.S77   1986   616.2'05   86-8387

ISBN: 0-671-60022-2

The author would like to acknowledge the assistance of R. Gordon Douglas, Jr., M.D., Professor and Chairman, Department of Medicine, Cornell University Medical College, and Physician-in-Chief, New York Hospital.

CONTENTS

1: THE COLD WAR

Does this sound familiar? You wake up one morning with a runny or stopped-up nose, a scratchy throat, and a funny feeling that all is not well with the world. You may have a fever, or you may feel chilled. You probably are sneezing, and you may have a cough. These symptoms *should* seem familiar. They are the classic signs of the common cold, the most common sickness known to humans.

Everyone catches colds. Each year, the average American adult comes down with two cases of the sniffles. Children under four years old get about eight colds a year. The dollar cost of this ailment is nothing to sneeze at. Americans spend about a billion dollars a year on medicines they hope will make them feel better. School children miss classes about sixty million days a year because of colds, and adults call in sick for almost fifty million days. Probably the most expensive colds on record took place on February 27, 1969. That was the night before the Apollo 9 spacecraft was scheduled to launch astronauts into orbit around the earth. All three astronauts showed up for work with cold symptoms. The National Aeronautics and Space Administration was forced to postpone the launch for a week. Those colds cost the United States government half a million dollars.

Some people get more colds than other people. Children are more prone than adults because their natural defenses against cold germs are less developed. After the age of three, girls are stricken more often than boys. In the teen years, girls get three colds a year, while boys average two. People who are upset by changes taking place in their lives get more colds than others. Even someone's personality affects the chances of catching the disease. Studies have shown that people who are shy get sick more often than people who are outgoing.

Some people assume that smoking cigarettes makes you more apt to come down with a cold. The truth is that smokers get the same number of colds as nonsmokers, but the colds they catch make them more miserable. Probably because smoking deposits unwanted particles in the lungs, smokers are more likely to get a hacking cough than people who stay away from cigarettes.

You can catch a cold any time of year, but you are most susceptible in the winter. The cold's close cousin, influenza (also called the flu) makes most of its attacks during the winter season, too. Cold weather does not seem to be the culprit, since one of the safest places in the world is the South Pole, where temperatures can fall to −100 degrees Fahrenheit. Scientists speculate that the cold and the flu spread most quickly during the winter because people spend a lot of time crowded indoors during these months. When people are close together, there is more opportunity for disease-causing germs to spread from one person to another. The South Pole is relatively safe because few people live there.

The very commonness of the cold makes it uncommon in the world of diseases. You probably will catch diseases like mumps or measles only once in your life, but you can expect to come down with colds over and over again. Why do people keep on catching colds? Why do colds spread so quickly? Why can't scientists, who have conquered hundreds of deadlier diseases, find a cure for the simple common cold? These are questions this book will answer.

THE SCENE OF THE CRIME

Cold germs like to settle in your nose and throat. The nose and throat form the upper respiratory tract*, a system of tubes that carries air to the lungs. When your nose is stuffy, you may have trouble breathing, but usually inhaling and exhaling air are quick, simple matters. Start to finish, the trip that air follows down the upper respiratory tract normally takes less than two-thirds of a second.

Air starts its journey in the nose or, much less often, the mouth. The nose is divided into two chambers, or nostrils, by a barrier called the septum. It is

*Defined in the glossary

11

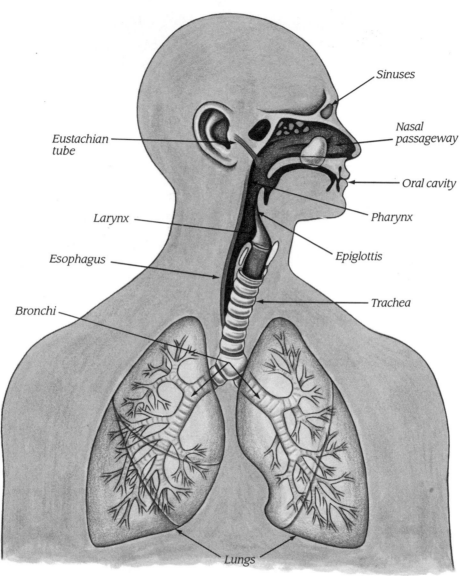

Sinuses

Nasal passageway

Eustachian tube

Oral cavity

Larynx

Pharynx

Esophagus

Epiglottis

Bronchi

Trachea

Lungs

The lungs draw down air from the atmosphere in less than two-thirds of a second.

made of rigid bone and a more flexible material known as cartilage*. In almost all people, the septum turns a bit to one side, making one nostril smaller than the other. The smaller nostril is more prone to becoming stuffed up than the larger one. Scientists have recently learned that the nostrils take turns inhaling. You breathe through one nostril for three to four hours, then switch to the other one.

From the nostrils, air travels through the nasal passageways to the pharynx*, the upper part of the throat. The mouth also leads into the pharynx. At this point, the air you breathe and the food you swallow travel in the same tube, a situation that soon changes. Just below the pharynx, the passageway branches into two tubes. One, the larynx*, or voice box, is a continuation of the air passageways. The voice box has a series of vibrating flaps, or vocal cords, with which you can turn air into speech.

The other tube, the esophagus*, leads to the stomach. When you swallow, a piece of cartilage called the epiglottis* swings shut over the airway and directs food and liquids to the esophagus. This area is the scene of many mishaps. If the epiglottis does not close at just the right moment, food goes down the wrong way. It gets into your air passages, causing coughing fits. The coughing forces the food back where it belongs.

The larynx leads to the trachea*, or windpipe. Near the bottom of the throat, the windpipe branches into two more tubes, the bronchi*. The bronchi enter the lower respiratory tract*, the right and left lungs. The bronchi then branch into increasingly smaller tubes, the bronchioles*.

This treelike structure of bronchioles ends in about 300 million alveoli*, or air sacs. Capillaries, very small vessels that carry blood, lie next to the alveoli. The air sacs absorb carbon dioxide from the blood in the capillaries. Carbon dioxide is a waste product the body needs to expel. This gas travels out of the lungs and up the respiratory tract, leaving your body by way of the mouth or nose.

Meanwhile, the capillaries absorb oxygen from the air sacs. The capillaries, now containing oxygen-rich blood, join a network of increasingly large blood vessels that lead to the left side of the heart. From the heart, the blood is pumped to every cell in the body. A process that begins in the nose or mouth ends up delivering needed oxygen throughout your body. In an adult, each day the respiratory system handles about five hundred cubic feet of air, about the amount contained in a large walk-in closet.

The upper respiratory tract does more than deliver air to and from the lungs. It also helps protect these very important organs. Your internal temperature is normally around 98.6 degrees Fahrenheit, but the air you breathe is usually much colder. Air heats up as it circulates in the nasal passageways and in the connecting sinuses, air-filled spaces in the skull. This warming system is very effective. If you breathe in air that is 10 degrees Fahrenheit, by the time it reaches the top of your throat, it will have heated up to 91 degrees.

Another important task of the upper respiratory tract is protecting your lungs from intruders. When you breathe, you pull in not only needed oxygen, but also unwelcome invaders like germs and dust particles. Your first line of defense against the intruders is the several hundred coarse hairs that stand guard at the entrance to the nostrils. They trap large particles and drops of moisture that can carry disease-causing germs.

Your second line of defense is the mucous membranes* that line the nasal passageways, sinuses, mouth, and upper throat. The mucous membranes contain blood vessels, nerve cells, and mucous cells. Mucous cells produce mucus*, the thick, sticky liquid that runs out of your nose. They also make an enzyme*, or chemical substance, that kills off some kinds of germs. When air passes over these membranes, the enzyme wipes out some germs and the mucus traps other intruders, keeping them away from the membranes.

Most of these membranes are lined with millions of tiny hairs called cilia. Invisible to the naked eye, these cilia beat backward and forward in waves, looking somewhat like the ripples you create in water when you row a boat. At a rate that can get up to one thousand beats a minute, the cilia move particle-laden mucus toward the back of the mouth. There, the mucus is swallowed, going down the esophagus and eventually entering the stomach. Acids in the stomach help kill off germs that are in the mucus.

Cilia are also present in the lower portion of the throat. Here, they push mucus away from the lungs and back up to the mouth where it is directed toward the stomach. Cilia beat at different speeds in different people. For the average person, it takes about ten minutes to move particles from the nostrils into the throat. For a slow-mover, the same trip may last

15

thirty minutes. Drinking alcohol or smoking tobacco produce chemical changes that may slow down the journey.

These defense systems work so well that the lungs are normally completely free of germs. Unfortunately, the upper respiratory tract is less efficient at protecting itself from disease. The mucous membranes that guard the lungs are precisely the spot where cold germs settle in.

A SNEAK ATTACK

Colds are silent attackers. You do not know that you have a cold until the germs have been entrenched in your upper respiratory tract for two to three days. At that time, the familiar, uncomfortable symptoms make an appearance.

You get sick from colds because they kill off some of the cells in your mucous membranes, but most of your misery comes from your body's attempt to fight back against the infection (see Chapter Three for more details). In its fight against the ailment, the body rushes blood to the nasal passages and sinuses, making them feel swollen. Healthy mucous cells produce more than normal amounts of mucus, giving you a runny nose. In children, the whole body gets involved in the fight by raising its temperature high enough to help kill germs. Adults rarely get feverish when they have colds.

Some organs not directly involved in breathing get in the path of the infection and show signs of illness, too. Colds may knock out the smelling organs inside your nose. Since what you taste is largely based on what you smell, colds can make meals seem bland and unappetizing. You have watery eyes with some colds because the disease can spread from your nasal passageways into the tear ducts that open into each eye. When you become hoarse or lose your voice, your larynx has also become infected.

People often mistake cold symptoms for those of the flu, or vice versa. Influenza symptoms are similar to cold symptoms, but they often go down deeper in the respiratory tract. Flu tends to strike very suddenly. You may feel fine in the morning, but by afternoon you feel as if you have been hit by a truck. Compared to a cold, a bout with the flu produces a higher fever, worse coughs, and more severe muscle aches. It usually takes longer to recover from the flu, often two to three weeks. The best way to tell if you have the flu or a cold is to look at what is happening to other people who live in your town. Influenza spreads more easily from person to person than colds do. If half the students in your school are in bed with the flu, chances are your symptoms are caused by the same disease. If you are the only sick person around, you probably have a cold.

Either way, flu or cold, infections that strike the upper respiratory tract can make you feel miserable. These infections, incidentally, start more often on Mondays than on any other day. Just who are the troublemakers who wreck a perfectly good week? In the next chapter, we will find out.

2: SPACE INVADERS

What causes the common cold and the flu? The names of these diseases do not give much of a hint. Colds, despite the name, do not come from standing in the cold. The flu does not come from the influence (*influenza* in Italian) of the stars, as seventeenth-century Italians believed. Scientists now know that these illnesses are caused by germs called viruses*.

Most infectious diseases – illnesses that spread from person to person – are due to either viruses or bacteria*. Bacteria, which are very simple, one-celled organisms, are usually visible under a standard light microscope, the type used in classrooms. Viruses, which are about a hundred times smaller than bacteria, cannot be seen with a standard microscope.

Medical experts suspected for

centuries that small infectious agents were responsible for many illnesses. In the 1870s the connection was firmly made. During those years, a French chemist named Louis Pasteur proved that bacteria-infected milk caused tuberculosis, a lung disease, in people. (The procedure he devised to kill bacteria in milk, called pasteurization, is still used today.) For the next few decades after Pasteur's discovery, researchers felt that bacteria were the only cause of contagious diseases. Then, around the turn of the century, a Dutch botanist named Martinus Willem Beijerinck challenged this idea through a famous experiment.

Beijerinck made a juice from tobacco leaves infected by the tobacco mosaic disease, which creates blotchy spots. He passed the juice through a piece of unglazed porcelain. The openings in porcelain were fine enough to filter out all the germs known at the time. Next the botanist rubbed the leaves of a healthy tobacco plant with the filtered juice. The plant came down with mosaic disease, proving that the ailment was caused by something smaller than bacteria. Beijerinck called the latest breed of germ a *virus*, which is Latin for "poison." In 1901, scientists first linked viruses to a disease found in humans, yellow fever. Now we know that these tiny germs are responsible for hundreds of diseases in people.

To get an idea of the size of a virus, picture an ant sitting on top of an elephant. Now imagine that elephant as the size of the point of a pin. A virus placed on the point of a pin looks like an ant on an elephant. Because of the smallness of viruses, scientists did not actually see them until the powerful electron microscope was invented in the 1940s. Under magnification several thousand times stronger than that with a standard microscope, viruses are rather beautiful. They are shaped like snowflakes or crystals.

Viruses are remarkable in another, more important, way. They are not quite alive. All living cells, including bacteria, can eat food, turn food into energy, move around, and reproduce, or make copies of themselves. Viruses can do none of these things on their own. They are incomplete agents, something like a car without an engine.

The outside of a virus is a protective protein shell. Inside, the main feature is some genetic material. A normal living cell contains two types of genetic information. DNA, short for dioxynucleic acid, provides the blueprints, or plans, for reproducing. It resembles a ladder twisted like a spiral staircase. RNA, short for ribonucleic acid, is like a building contractor. Using the information provided by DNA, it directs the building of new proteins. In a normal cell, both kinds of nucleic acid pitch in to create new cells.

Viruses contain either RNA or DNA, never both. Consequently, left to their own devices, they cannot reproduce. They lie dormant for years, possibly centuries, and come to "life" only when they latch onto living cells.

SMALL SABOTEURS

Here is how a virus does its damage. First, the virus attaches itself to the outside membrane of a healthy cell. Then it penetrates the cell. Once inside, it somehow takes over the reproductive tools of the cell. It directs the cell to produce not new cells, but new viruses. This

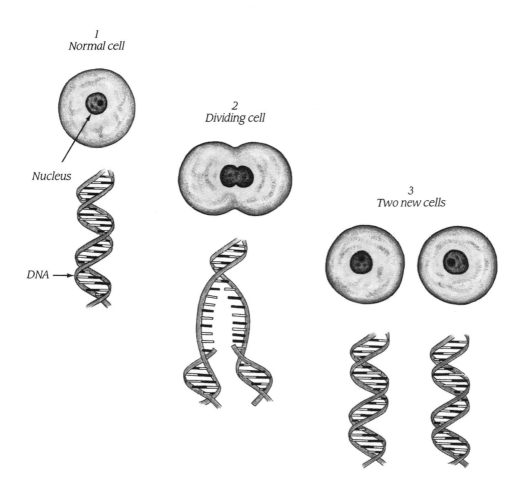

1
Normal cell

Nucleus

DNA →

2
Dividing cell

3
Two new cells

How a cell normally reproduces.

Shaped like a coiled ladder, DNA contains the information needed for a cell to make a copy of itself. When a cell reproduces, it forms a second nucleus, or center, then splits in half. The DNA inside the nucleus splits down the middle, forming two half-ladders (2). Each "rung" in the half-ladders picks up fragments lying around in the nucleus. The resulting two ladders (3) are exact replicas of the original one (1). RNA in the nucleus directs the whole reproduction operation, giving instructions to the dividing cell based on the information contained in DNA.

21

is something like an army officer marching into a bicycle factory and telling the workers to make tanks instead of bikes. The cell complies with the orders, producing several thousand "daughter" viruses in a few minutes to a few hours. The host cell then releases the new viruses, either slowly over the space of several hours, or quickly all in one rush. These new viruses are now free to attack other living cells. The original host cell becomes weakened by its superhuman production effort, separates from its neighboring cells, and dies.

Viruses are dangerous because they can kill cells. Bacteria are responsible for the death of cells, too, but in a different way. With bacteria, a toxin, or poison, is usually the murder weapon. Sometimes these toxins are by-products of bacterial cell reproduction. At other times, the toxins come from cells the human body produces to fight off invaders.

Viruses are choosy about their victims. They seem to stay away from snakes, yeasts, shellfish, and cone-bearing evergreens, but thrive in birds and mammals. The outer protective coating of viruses is programmed to hook onto certain kinds of cells, somewhat like keys designed to fit only into particular locks. Some virologists, people who study viruses, feel that this made-to-order quality of viruses gives a clue to their origin. The scientists speculate that viruses evolved from working parts of cells that somehow "escaped" but periodically "return home" and live off other organisms.

The more important the cells that a virus attacks, the more serious the resulting disease is. The rabies virus, which can attack brain cells, is a bigger threat than a cold virus, which

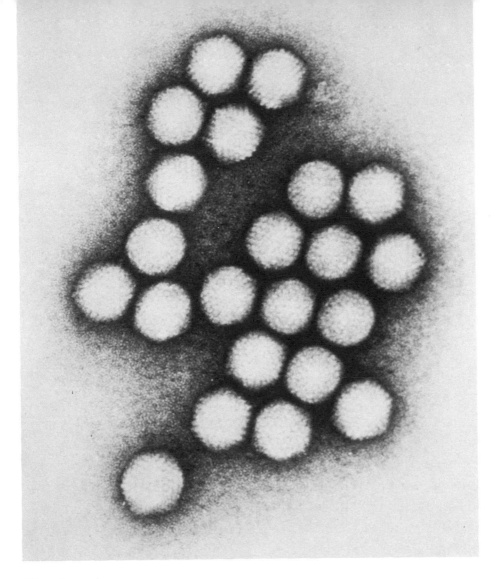

The adeno virus.
In the 1950s and 1960s, researchers learned that the cold many American army recruits developed in training camp came from two forms of the adeno virus. By 1971, a vaccine was developed against these two viruses. Now, all army recruits take two vaccine pills during their first twenty-four hours of training camp. The vaccine has made the incidence of adeno virus-caused colds drop by half in these camps.

23

overpowers cells in the upper respiratory tract. You can afford to lose a lot more tissue, or collections of cells, in your nose than in your brain. Similarly, influenza viruses are more dangerous than cold viruses because, unlike cold viruses, flu viruses can destroy cells in your lungs.

Many people wonder why viral infections are more difficult to beat back than bacterial infections. With bacterial infections like tuberculosis, typhoid fever, and strep throat, antibiotic medicines are usually effective in killing off the infectious agents. These drugs kill off bacteria by interfering with their ability to reproduce and make energy. Since viruses do not perform these functions unless they are inside a cell, it is usually not possible to destroy a virus without killing an infected cell. Only a very few medicines exist that can harm viruses without harming their host cells (see Chapter Five).

HOW VIRUSES GET AROUND

Viruses have many traits in common, but they vary greatly in size, shape, and how they act. For instance, nucleic acid makes up only 1 percent of the contents of an influenza virus, but 25 percent of a polio virus and 50 percent of viruses that attack bacteria. The variety is similar to that found within the animal kingdom. Two kinds of viruses may resemble each other only as much as a snake is similar to a human being.

Over two hundred different kinds of viruses cause the common cold. Despite their differences, they produce similar symptoms in human beings. The two most important families of cold-causing viruses are the

24

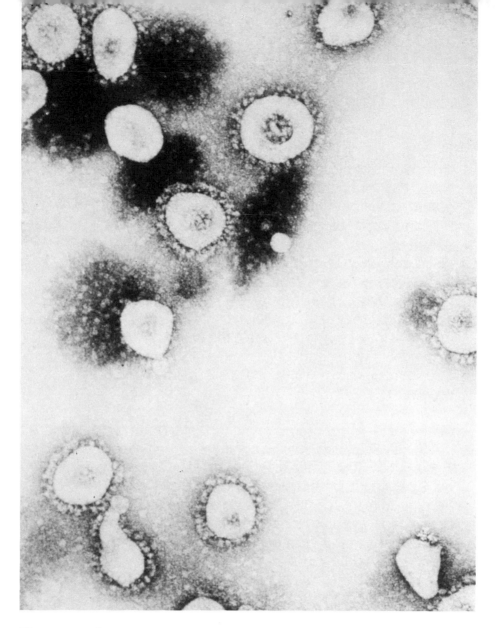

The corona virus.
The second largest cause of colds, corona viruses have a halolike "corona," or crown. These viruses usually cause colds during the winter, often affecting large parts of a community at the same time.

25

The Cold Front

In 1946, British scientists decided to turn an empty hospital into the world's only research institution devoted to the study of the common cold. The research center, called the Common Cold Unit, is located in attractive countryside about ninety miles outside of London, England. Each year, hundreds of British men and women stay at the center for ten-day periods and try to catch colds. Because the government pays their expenses, plus a little pocket money, some couples even spend their vacations here. These trips are an endless source of amusement to British comedians. All research at the center is done on humans, since the only animals that come down with people-type colds are chimpanzees. Chimpanzees are too mischievous to follow doctors' orders.

Some years ago, the Common Cold Unit decided to test, once and for all, the common belief that getting cold gives you colds. Scientists divided volunteers into three groups. People in the first group received nose drops containing cold-causing viruses. Then they stood in dripping wet bathing suits in a chilly room for half an hour. The second group of people also received the drops, but did nothing else unusual. A third group of people underwent the wet bathing suit routine, but did not get drops. A few days later, scientists learned that people who had not been exposed to cold germs did not catch colds, even if they had been shivering for a half hour. The people exposed to the germs did catch cold. Those who shivered got no more colds than those who did not. The moral of this story is that being cold does not give you a cold. The situation is really the opposite. Having a cold makes you feel cold, or chilly.

rhino virus and the corona virus. Together, these families cause about half of all colds. Rhino viruses, named for the Greek word for "nose," strike most in the fall and winter. Corona viruses are responsible for many summer colds. They are crownlike circles, resembling the corona, or halo, sometimes seen around the sun. Six other virus families are known to cause about 10 percent of colds. The precise cause of the remaining 40 percent of sniffles is still a mystery.

Recent research says that cold viruses are passed from person to person mainly through the hands, not the air. Cold viruses enter the body mostly by way of the nose or the tear ducts in the eyes. If you touch something that has been touched by an infected person, then rub your eyes or nose, you conveniently drop off cold viruses at the spots where they feel most welcome.

3: THE BODY STRIKES BACK

The body does not take invasion by outsiders lying down. When intruders get by the barriers in the upper respiratory tract (see Chapter One), the body calls upon its army of defenders, known as the immune system. The immune system takes swift, sure action, helping us recover from a cold or the flu within a few days or weeks. The immune system also looks out for our future health by providing protection or immunity from later attacks by the same intruders.

The very first defensive maneuver happens just three to four hours after a host cell is invaded. The host cell cannot stop the attacking virus from taking over its workings, but it can sabotage takeovers of other cells. An attack causes the host cell to produce a substance known as interferon*. This substance is released by the dying cell into the fluids that surround it. Interferon contains a chemical message that alerts nearby cells about the impending attack. The alerted cells then make an antiviral protein. When an attacking virus penetrates these alerted cells, they have the power to disobey the commands of the virus. These cells continue to create cells in their own image rather than viruses. Interferon is released from infected cells hours before these cells release new viruses. This substance is thus able to delay an invasion by viruses, creating a holding action until the big guns of the immune system are able to reach the scene.

ATTACK OF THE WHITE BLOOD CELLS

White blood cells are the most powerful weapon in the body's defense arsenal. Colorless rather than white, these cells are born in bone marrow, may mature elsewhere, and are then transported around the body via the bloodstream or the drainage system known as the lymphatic system* They tend to gather in the lymph nodes in your body, especially those in your neck, armpits, or groin. When you have an infection, so much activity goes on in these lymph nodes that they often become sore and swollen. Sometimes you know you are sick because you can feel these swollen glands in your neck.

Red blood cells carry oxygen to cells throughout the body. White blood cells, which are outnumbered five hundred to one by the red variety, perform a much bigger variety of tasks. Their main functions are to kill off invaders and to get rid of ill or dead cells. The pus that forms in an infected cut is partly made up of white blood cells that fight off bacteria.

The first type of white blood cell to show up at the scene of an attack is a large cell known as a macrophage*, or "big eater." This scavenger is an all-purpose weapon. During the early phase of an infection, the big eater wanders around the body until it blindly bumps into an intruder. Once it hooks onto an intruder, it flows around and surrounds the foreigner. Then it shoots out a balloon of digestive enzymes that break the intruder apart. With its voracious appetite, a big eater can consume up to a hundred viruses before it too dies.

The big eater gets back-up support from a type of white blood cell called a lymphocyte*. Smaller and rounder than macrophages, lymphocytes are tailor-made to fight very specific enemies. Because of this made-to-order quality, they can make a beeline for the specific intruders that are causing the infection. Lymphocytes are a much more powerful weapon against invading viruses than are big eaters.

Lymphocytes come in two forms, T cells and B cells. With infections that do not last long, like colds and bouts of the flu, T cells are the more important weapon. T cells start out in bone marrow, but are "trained" in the thymus, a small gland underneath the upper part of the breastbone. As part of their education, T cells learn to respond to cells infected with one type of invader. Each T cell has a receptor, a spot on its outside membrane that makes it sensitive to the chemical makeup of a certain intruder. The variety of T cells is enormous. Out of a hundred thousand T cells, for instance, only one may be able to spot a mucous membrane cell invaded by a particular cold-causing virus.

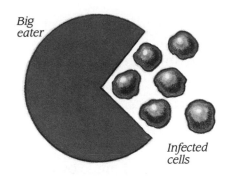

Big
eater

Infected
cells

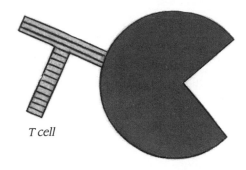

T cell

Killer
T cells

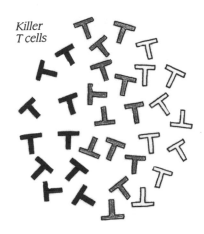

Killer T cells attacking
infected cells

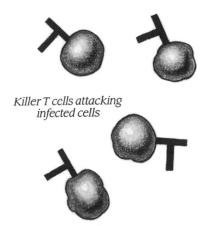

Stemming the spread of infection.

*Like a Pac Man, the big eater (1) gobbles up cells that have been infected with
cold viruses. The activity draws the attention of special cells known as T cells (2).
The big eater relays the identifying markers of the virus to the T cells. The few T
cells that recognize this marker send out messages calling in more troops to fight
the virus. These T cells also produce four types of daughter cells (3) in great
numbers. One of these daughter cells, the killer T cell (4), then sets out after
other infected cells. When killer T cells find infected cells, they send out a poison
that dissolves these cells, which prevents viruses from spreading.*

B cells have even more specialized weapons at their disposal. While T cells act only against infected human cells, B cells, when given the right information, are able to produce antibodies* that neutralize specific invaders. The B cells can make these refined weapons because they have "jumping genes." The gene in the B cell that makes antibodies comes in about seven separate pieces. These can move around to create an enormous number of different antibodies, each tailored to a different antigen*, or invader.

Antibodies neutralize viruses by blocking their surfaces so they can no longer attach to the cells they are keyed to. Since it takes the body about two weeks to make antibodies, these weapons usually are not built in time to stop a cold or flu infection. The ones that get built, however, are an investment in the future. They patrol your bloodstream, ready to disarm any viruses attempting to make return visits. These sentries are also partially effective at neutralizing new invaders that are fairly similar to ones you have already battled against.

For a fairly minor infection like a cold or the flu, the battle against the invaders takes place in the following way. First, big eaters happen upon the scene, gobbling up infected cells and viruses. Hordes of T cells and some B cells follow. The T cells touch against the big eaters, picking up a chemical signal that identifies the form of the invader. The very few T cells that are sensitive to this signal react by sending out chemical messages for reinforcements. One of these messages, in a form of interferon, turns the big eaters into faster-than-normal gobblers.

The sensitive T cells also

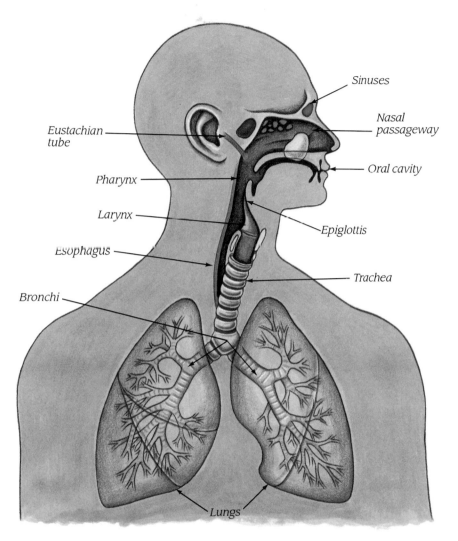

Sinuses

Nasal passageway

Oral cavity

Eustachian tube

Pharynx

Larynx

Esophagus

Epiglottis

Trachea

Bronchi

Lungs

When all systems are A-OK, it takes less than two-thirds of a second to draw air from the atmosphere down to your lungs, a journey of about sixteen inches in an adult. The first leg of the trip usually begins in the nasal passageway, where air flows around for about a quarter of a second. Air then passes through the pharynx (upper throat) and larynx (voice box) in less than one-tenth of a second. Warmed and moistened in the earlier legs of the trip, air now travels through the trachea (windpipe) and the two branching bronchi within a third of a second. The bronchi lead the air to its final destinations, the right and left lungs.

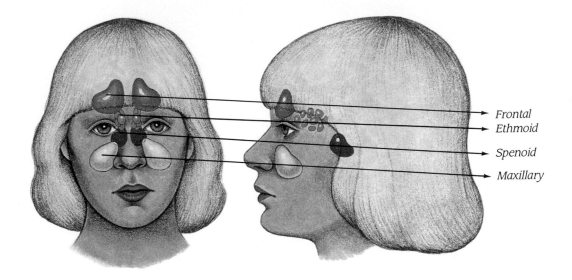

Frontal
Ethmoid
Spenoid
Maxillary

The bones in the front of your head form four sets of air-filled spaces known as sinuses. When you have a cold, the mucous membranes lining the sinuses can become infected and inflamed. The sinus cavities most prone to infection are the frontal and maxillary ones. If you have an infection in the frontal sinuses, you usually get a headache. Inflammation of the maxillary sinuses may give you pain around your cheekbones.

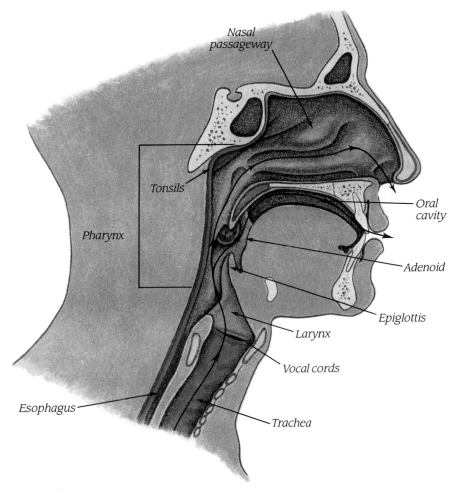

Nasal passageway

Tonsils

Pharynx

Oral cavity

Adenoid

Epiglottis

Larynx

Vocal cords

Esophagus

Trachea

How you talk.

Just before you talk, you quickly inhale air through the nose. Then you exhale air out of the lungs, up the trachea, through the larynx, home of the vocal cords. The vocal cords are two bands of cartilage attached to muscles in the larynx. They are somewhat like curtains that open or close at your command. When you are not talking, the curtains are open. When you wish to speak, you shut the curtains partway. Air traveling through partly closed vocal cords causes the cords to vibrate, which makes noise. A cold or the flu can temporarily change your voice. If your larynx becomes infected, your vocal cords may not work right, and you may become hoarse or even lose your voice.

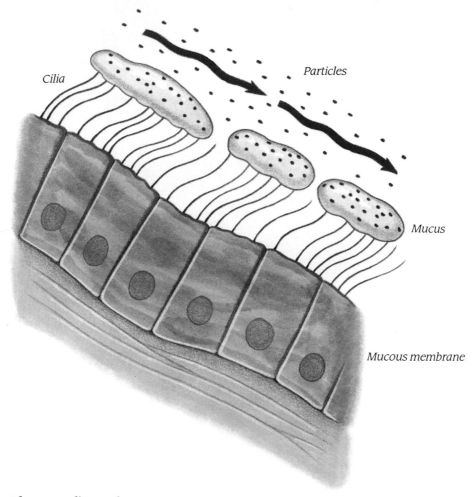

Cilia

Particles

Mucus

Mucous membrane

The germ disposal system.
Tiny particles that make it past the nose's first line of defense, the nasal hairs, come up against a second trap, mucus. Clumps of germ-grabbing mucus rest on top of the cilia that grow out of mucous membranes. The cilia, beating in unison, push the mucus toward the throat. After you swallow the mucus, it and whatever it contains are destroyed by stomach juices.

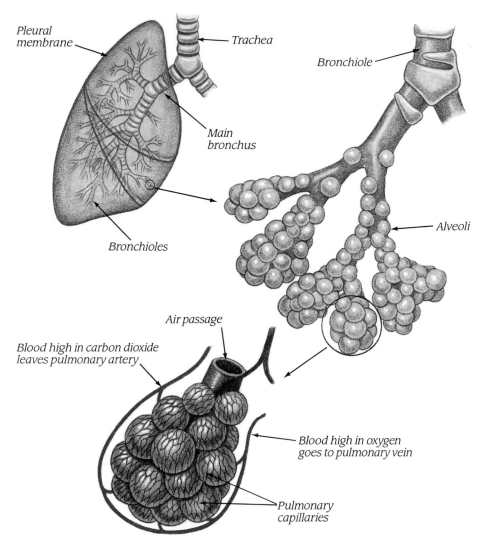

Pleural membrane

Trachea

Bronchiole

Main bronchus

Alveoli

Bronchioles

Air passage

Blood high in carbon dioxide leaves pulmonary artery

Blood high in oxygen goes to pulmonary vein

Pulmonary capillaries

The lungs at work.

Surrounded by the pleural membrane, which acts like a cushion, the lungs are made up of increasingly smaller air passages. Air reaches the lungs by means of the trachea (1), which splits into two main bronchi. The bronchi, in turn, branch into smaller bronchioles (2). The smallest bronchioles are like dead-end streets. They terminate in air sacs. These air sacs, or alveoli, are covered with a network of capillaries, very tiny blood vessels (3). These capillaries drop off their load of carbon dioxide at the air sacs, then pick up a supply of oxygen. The high-oxygen blood is then shipped towards the heart, which distributes it throughout the body.

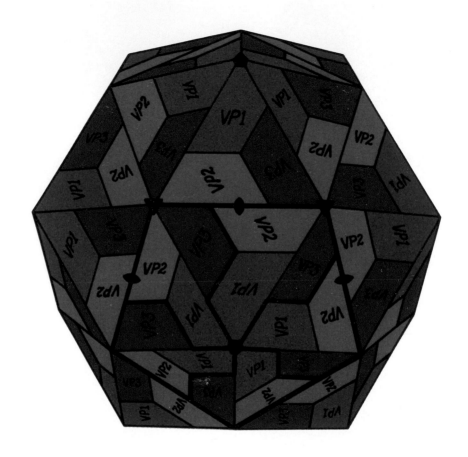

Using complicated computer procedures, scientists have recently built a map of the rhino virus, the most common cause of the cold. Like all viruses, the rhino virus has a crystal structure. The sections VP1, VP2, and VP3 on the map are different proteins that make up the outside of the virus.

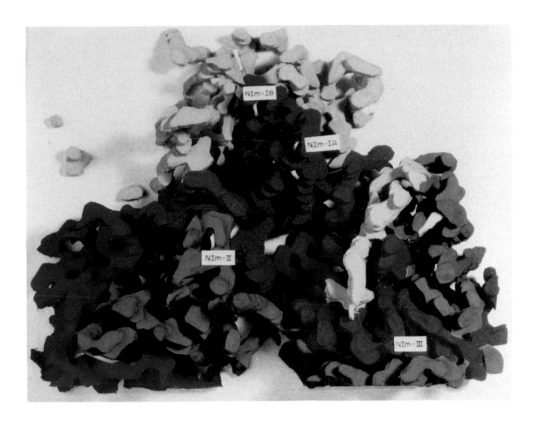

This model made of balsa wood shows a small section of the exterior of the rhino virus. The protein VP1 is light and dark blue, VP2 is green, and VP3 is red. The portions labeled NIm-IA, NIm-IB, NIm-II, and NIm-III are spots that stimulate the production of human antibodies against the virus.

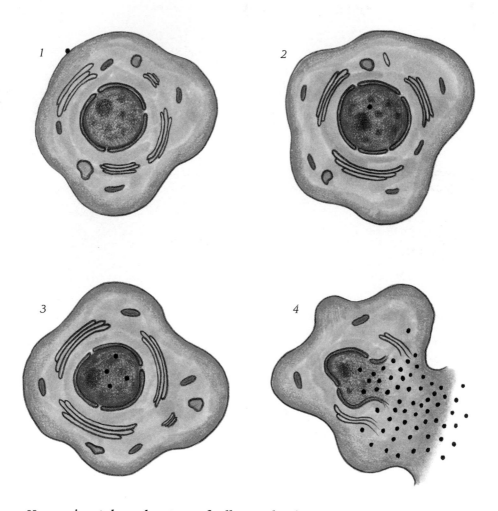

How a virus takes advantage of cell reproduction.
(1) A virus attaches itself to the outside membrane of a healthy cell. It moves toward the center of the cell and (2) seems to become engulfed. The virus frees itself of the cell's membrane and takes over the reproductive machinery, rapidly producing new "daughter" viruses. (3) These viruses leave the cell (4) and search for new victims. The once-healthy cell pulls apart from the tissue it is attached to and dies.

react by dividing into massive numbers of four new types of T cells, all designed to deal with the specific invader. The most important daughter cell, the killer T, can kill cells infected with the virus. Another daughter, the helper T, assists B cells in producing antibodies. A third cell, the suppressor T, tells all the other T cells when to stop their activities. Finally, the memory T stores information about the intruder for future reference. Most mature lymphocyte cells live for only a short time, but memory ones go on for decades. Like wizened village elders, they remember the details of old wars. When the same enemy returns, they tell the young warriors how the intruder was vanquished in times gone by.

By preventing viruses from reproducing and by killing off some of the actual intruders, the main soldiers in the immune system – interferon, big eaters, and lymphocytes – almost always get you over an attack by a cold or flu virus.

WHY YOU FEEL SICK

Your upper respiratory tract may be the scene of a violent battle for days before you realize you have caught a cold. The symptoms of a cold, what makes you feel ill, are largely the result of a mechanism that helps white blood cells rush to the scene of the action. This mechanism, inflammation*, usually starts within a few days after you have been infected. Until the inflammation begins, the attack has generally been painless.

Infection by viruses in the upper respiratory tract causes specialized cells in the mucous membranes to release a powerful chemical called histamine. Histamine makes the walls of nearby tiny blood

33

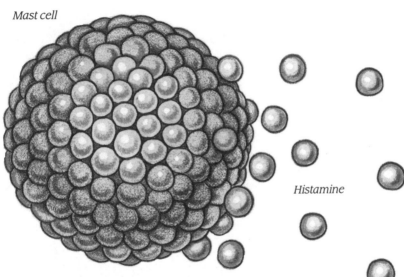

Mast cell

Histamine

Why your nose gets runny.
Stimulated by infection, specialized cells in the nasal membranes, called mast cells, produce several powerful chemicals. One of them, known as histamine, lands in special receptors on the walls of nearby arterioles, very small arteries. Once in the receptors, histamine causes the muscles in the walls to expand. This expansion allows more blood to flow to the area. It also causes liquid in the blood vessel to seep into nasal tissue. Swollen by the seeping liquid, the nasal tissues become narrow, or congested, making you feel stuffy. Mucus that normally flows through these passages cannot get by and instead runs out your nose.

34

vessels, called arterioles, dilate, or expand. The expansion means that more blood can reach the infected area. Dilation also stretches the walls of the blood vessels. The effect is similar to what happens when you pull on a sock. Spaces between the cells that make up the vessel walls become larger. The enlarged spaces allow infection-fighting agents and fluids in the bloodstream to seep out into the mucous membranes. This fluid makes the membranes swell, which in turn causes the nasal passages to narrow. The feeling of stuffiness and congestion you get with a cold is due to this swelling. Congestion does not mean, as many people think, that your nose has become clogged with mucus.

Attempting to sweep invaders out of the area, mucous membranes do produce more mucus. Your nose may start running because this extra mucus cannot get through your narrowed nasal passages. Meanwhile, the swollen membranes press against sensitive nerve endings, shooting pain signals to the brain. These signals may give you a sore nose and a headache. The swelling may also send messages to the sneeze center in the brain. The sneeze center instructs muscles around the lungs to contract suddenly, causing an explosion of air to leave the mouth and, to a lesser extent, the nose. This explosion, going at a speed of up to a hundred miles an hour, temporarily clears your nasal cavities of extra mucus.

Similarly, swelling and irritation may stimulate the cough center in the brain to help clear out the throat and lungs. A cough happens when the chest and stomach muscles tighten and the epiglottis at the top of the larynx closes. Pressure builds up inside the lungs because the closed larynx prevents air from getting out. The epiglottis then suddenly opens, somewhat like a balloon that bursts when it is filled with too much air. Trapped air is released by the lungs in a burst that can reach five hundred miles an hour.

For children, a common side effect in colds and the flu is fever. When you have a fever, or a higher-than-normal temperature, your internal temperature regulator has become turned up. As with the thermostat in a house, when your own thermostat goes higher, you are producing more energy. Your body-building mechanisms have shot into high speed. You are burning up your food faster than usual, you are breathing quickly, and your heart is pumping swiftly.

Oddly, sometimes when you have a fever, you feel chilled. That is because your thermostat is calling for a higher temperature than you have reached. You feel chilled not because you are cold, but because you are falling short of the aimed-for temperature. Shivering, all-over contractions in the muscles, is your body's way to make extra heat. The contractions warm you up just as running around the block does. At high temperatures (102 degrees Fahrenheit for an adult, 103 degrees for a child), a fever seriously endangers your health. You risk "cooking" your internal organs. Lower fevers, however, may help you. Some scientists feel that moderately high temperatures make your body's white blood cells more effective at fending off invasions. Also, the speeding up of production that comes with fevers helps you quickly make your best allies.

4: THE FLU— A DEADLIER CASE

An epidemic is the spread of an infectious disease in a large but well-defined area, such as a state. A pandemic is a worldwide spread that affects millions of people. Influenza is the only remaining pandemic disease on earth. Modern science has conquered all the others.

The worst outbreak of influenza occurred during the years 1918 and 1919. The Japanese called this particular strain the American flu, the Chinese called it the Japanese flu, but most of the world knows it as the Spanish flu. By conservative estimates, one-fifth of the human race alive at the time suffered from the aches and fever of the ailment. About twenty million people worldwide died from the disease, or, more accurately, from its complications.

Complications are diseases caused by another disease. In the United States, at least half a million people were killed by the Spanish flu.

Normally, the flu strikes most people in a community, but is fatal only to the very young and the very old. The Spanish flu was different. Unlike any strain of influenza before or since 1918 and 1919, this version mainly struck down people who were in the prime of their lives. In San Francisco, California, for instance, two-thirds of the people who died as a result of the flu were between the ages of twenty and forty. Statistics were similar in other cities.

Throughout the world, life ground to a halt in some places. All over the country, schools, churches, theaters, and saloons shut down. The Bell Telephone Company of Pennsylvania was so low on staff that it posted a sign requesting customers to make "only absolutely necessary calls compelled by the epidemic or by war necessity." (This was during World War I.) Volunteers visited the sick, tended orphaned children, and brought food to stricken families.

People took some desperate, and useless, precautions against the infection. The Commissioner of Health in New York State made it illegal for anyone to cough or sneeze in public without covering his or her face with a handkerchief. *The New York Times* reported some advice from the New York City Commissioner of Health. The commissioner suggested that "any fellow kissing a girl would be wise to do it through a handkerchief."

In some U.S. towns, children wore bags filled with the strong-smelling chemical camphor around their necks. The camphor fumes were thought to knock out the "bug." Gauze face masks covered faces from Sydney, Australia, to Calgary, Canada, to Shanghai, China. It was hoped that the masks would filter out flu germs. Unfortunately, these bags and masks did little or nothing to stop the spread of influenza.

After three waves of infection, the Spanish flu ultimately lost its power in 1919. Scientists rank this pandemic with the Black Plague, which decimated the population of Europe in the fourteenth century, as one of the great killer diseases of history. No flu pandemic since that time has equaled this disease. Lesser pandemics, however, still tend to strike every ten to twenty years. In 1957, for instance, more than forty-five million Americans came down with the Asian flu. Over fifty thousand people in the United States died from it. During the most recent pandemic, in the winter of 1968

to 1969, the Hong Kong flu struck one-quarter of the American population, and killed about thirty thousand people. In nonpandemic years, the flu is still a significant cause of illness and death. When the flu is milder, about 10 to 20 percent of the U.S. population catches it. People most likely to die from it are the very old and people with chronic diseases such as heart disease, kidney trouble, or lung problems.

The Spanish flu is still one of the great mysteries of modern science. Medical experts do not know why it spread so quickly or why it was deadly to people in their middle years. Efforts to track down the precise virus have failed. The most energetic attempt occurred in 1951, when a team of scientists traveled to Alaska to dig up bodies of Spanish flu victims. They found several well-preserved bodies in the Arctic tundra, but were not able to isolate viable flu viruses from the lung tissues. The best guess of scientists now is that the Spanish flu resembles a virus currently found in swine.

THE NATURE OF THE CULPRIT

Until 1918, scientists believed that influenza was caused by bacteria. Autopsies of victims failed to support this theory of bacterial infection. Then, in 1930, the first influenza virus was discovered in swine. Three years later, the first human flu virus was tracked down. This virus came to be called influenza A. A second form, influenza B, was found in 1940. The third type, influenza C, was identified in 1947.

Influenza A is the most severe form. It occurs in a variety of animals, notably swine, birds, and horses, while B and C seem to show up only in humans. Only influenza A causes pandemics. The B form causes milder epidemics that are more of a danger for children than for adults. Influenza C is not a significant cause of illness. Influenza pandemics and epidemics appear in the winter months (between November and March in the Northern Hemisphere), but individual cases can occur at any season.

The inner core of an influenza virus contains genetic material. This genetic material is arranged in an unusual way for viruses that live in animals. The RNA in a flu virus comes in eight separate pieces, while for most viruses the genetic package is one strand. Each time a flu virus reproduces, the eight new genes must line up the way the genes in the original virus did in order for the new virus to become an exact copy of the first one. Because the genes are separate, there is more chance for mishaps to occur than with

40

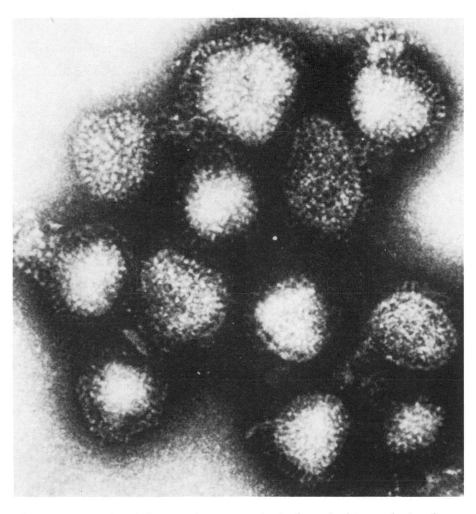

This type A "Russian" influenza virus was active in the United States during the mid-1970s. It is magnified here thousands of times by an electron microscope.

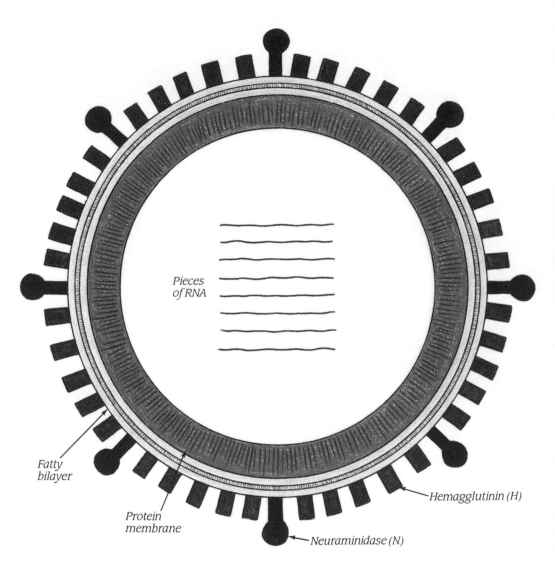

Pieces
of RNA

Fatty
bilayer

Protein
membrane

Hemagglutinin (H)

Neuraminidase (N)

Diagram of a flu virus.
The joint efforts of the hemagglutinin (H) and neuraminidase (N) spikes get the flu virus inside a respiratory cell. The spikes are anchored in two layers of fat, which cover a protein membrane. Inside are eight separate pieces of RNA. In most viruses, including cold viruses, RNA is a continuous strand.

most viruses. This means that the rate of mutation, or chance variation, is higher in flu viruses than in other kinds of viruses.

From the point of view of the human immune system, the most important mutations are those that occur in the outer surface of a flu virus. Each time a human cell is infected with a virus, the body produces antibodies that act against the proteins on its outer surface. The next time a person is infected with that virus, the antibodies head off a new viral infection. If the virus changes its form, however, the existing antibodies are not as useful in providing protection. The greater the change in the virus's surface characteristics, the less useful these antibodies are.

For an influenza A virus, the most common type, the human body produces antibodies against two forms of spikes that appear on the outer surface of the virus. One spike is called hemagglutinin (H)*. The name comes from its tendency to combine with red blood cells and cause them to agglutinate*, or clump. The H spike of an influenza virus matches proteins on the outer surface of respiratory cells. This match allows the virus to pick the correct host cell.

The second spike is called neuraminidase (N)*. The N spike is an enzyme, or chemical activator. It dissolves the linkage between the H spike and red blood cells. If the link were not dissolved, the virus would be part of a clump too large to squeeze into a cell. The N spike also seems to help "daughter" viruses get out of an infected cell. A swine flu virus contains around five hundred H spikes and one hundred N spikes. The H spikes in influenza A viruses appear to mutate more often than the N spikes. These mutations pave the way for epidemics and pandemics.

How A New Strain Is Born

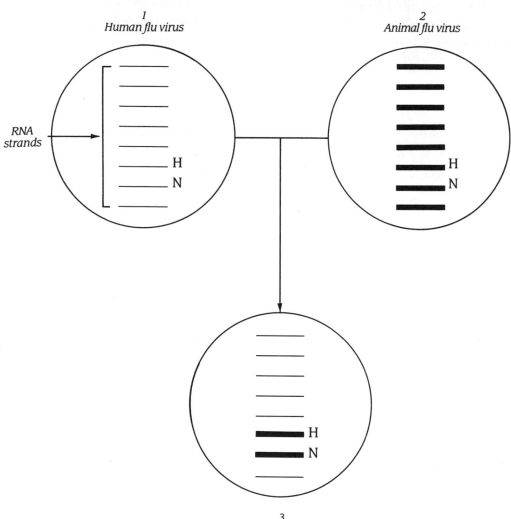

1
Human flu virus

2
Animal flu virus

RNA
strands

H
N

H
N

H
N

3
Human-infecting hybrid

Every ten or twenty years a completely new strain of influenza virus emerges. Since no one has immunity to this virus, it tends to sweep the earth, causing a worldwide pandemic. One theory as to how these new strains come about suggests that they start in animals, especially birds. Inside virus-laden cells of an animal, two flu viruses crossbreed. One is a virus that can infect humans, the other is a virus that invades only animals. The product of the crossbreeding is a virus that takes from the human form the ability to reproduce inside humans. From the animal form it gets new H and N spikes. Since humans have never before encountered these H and N spikes, they have no antibodies to protect them against the hybrid virus.

Besides its greater ability to change, the flu virus has one other quality that makes it more contagious than cold viruses. Flu viruses travel more easily through the air than cold viruses. After a sneeze or cough, cold germs can journey in the air only on fairly large droplets of water. Flu viruses can hitch a ride on very small droplets as well. These droplets, too small for a gauze mask to filter out, tend to stay in the air for long periods of time. You can pick up a flu virus by sitting in a movie theater where, an hour earlier, an infected person coughed. You would probably not catch a cold this way. Fortunately, scientists are coming up with ways to fend off the flu that are more effective than wearing face masks.

5: TAKING CARE OF YOURSELF

There is an old adage, "Treat a cold and it will last a week, do nothing and it will go away in seven days." The saying is as true now as it was a hundred years ago. At present, no cold remedy is able to prevent, cure, or shorten the length of a cold. Remedies can make you feel better, but they do not fight against the viruses that are the cause of the sickness.

The simplest way to treat a cold is to get rest and to drink plenty of liquids. Most doctors agree that if you feel like slowing down because of a cold, you should. If you do not feel like taking it easy, then don't. Drinking liquids such as fruit juice helps loosen mucus that has become stuck in your upper respiratory tract. They soothe a dry, sore throat. They also help replace water lost through perspiration if you have a fever. Milk is not a good option for some people. It tends to make you produce more mucus. At Mount Sinai Medical Center in Miami Beach, Florida, researchers found that drinking hot water or chicken soup speeds up the rate at which mucus leaves the nasal passages. Vapors from the hot liquids give the process a boost.

In 1972, the Food and Drug Administration, the government agency that oversees drugs, called together an expert panel. The panel's task was to evaluate the safety and effectiveness of various over-the-counter, or nonprescription, cold remedies. The panel's recommendations were meant for adults.

The panel recommended against using products that treat more than one symptom at once. For instance, some pills are for both runny noses and fevers. The trouble is, you are not likely to have several symptoms at once, or even with the same bout of the cold. The extra medicine is unnecessary. You can tell which symptoms a medicine treats by looking at the claims on the package. The symptoms that cold medicines are good for, according to the panel, are runny or congested noses, coughs, and aches and pains. Many doctors who take care of children believe that cold medicines are not good for children.

A nasal decongestant can sometimes help to clear up a stuffy nose, the panel concluded. The panel felt that two other classes of drugs, antihistamines* and anticholinergics*, are not effective for simple colds. Nasal decongestants in nose drops and sprays constrict enlarged blood vessels in the nasal passages. If they are used for too

47

long a time or too often, however, they have a rebound effect. That is, they begin to enlarge rather than constrict the blood vessels, making your nose feel even more stuffed.

Coughs come in two varieties. "Productive" coughs are those that bring mucus up out of the throat, helping unclog the upper respiratory tract. "Nonproductive" coughs result when inflammation in the throat stimulates the muscular cough reflex. They do not help, and can seriously irritate the throat. Cough medicines deal with coughs in different ways. Antitussives* chemically suppress the cough center in the brain, while expectorants* are intended to thin mucus so it can more easily leave bronchial airways. According to the FDA panel, antitussives are effective workers, but expectorants do not do their job. Again, many doctors don't recommend cough medicines for children because of their side effects and their questionable value. For coughs that need just a little boost, drinking a hot liquid or sucking on a hard candy helps loosen up mucus a bit.

For aches and pains or fever, most doctors recommend aspirin, or the aspirin substitute acetaminophen. Some version of aspirin has been around for almost two thousand years, but only in 1971 did scientists discover why it helps relieve pain. Aspirin inhibits the production of body chemicals that cause, among other things, inflammation. Since inflammation of the mucous membranes is the chief source of discomfort during a cold, aspirin brings effective relief. A similar drug, ibuprofen (marketed as Advil or Nuprin), was recently made available as an over-the-counter drug. Not recommended for children, ibuprofen inhibits the same chemicals as aspirin.

When it comes to a sore throat, drugstore medications are not much help. The FDA has determined that throat lozenges are not effective in soothing angry throats. A more effective treatment is to gargle with warm water mixed with ordinary salt.

Is there any way to prevent the misery of a cold? One way to reduce your chances of picking up viruses is to wash your hands frequently and to avoid putting your fingers near your eyes and nose. Many scientists also believe that eating foods packed with vitamins and minerals helps you fight off infections. You need these micronutrients in certain amounts to keep your body functions, including your immune system, in tip-top shape. Some people go a step further. They think that taking megadoses, or much larger than normal doses, of specific micronutrients will give you extra protection against colds and flu.

In 1970, Dr. Linus Pauling, a Stanford University chemist, published a book called *Vitamin C and the Common Cold*. Pauling put forth the view that megadoses of vitamin C, some 150 times higher than the government recommends, stop people from getting colds. Although a few experiments have supported his view, the evidence is that there is no reason to take more vitamin C than the recommended level. The body excretes excess doses. What you end up with, in the words of one researcher, is nothing more than "very expensive urine."

In 1985, another micronutrient was touted as a cold-stopper. A Texas man, not a doctor, thought that sucking on tablets containing the mineral zinc

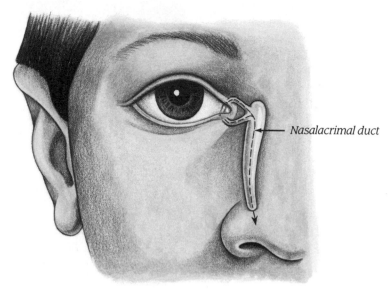

Nasalacrimal duct

The nose/eye connection.
Rub your eye after you have touched something infected with a cold virus, and you will put the virus in its favorite spot, the nose. Why? Because a passageway called the nasalacrimal duct connects the inside corner of the eye to the nose. (You can see the opening in the corner of your eye if you look closely.) The tube normally drains away extra tears. These tears constantly wash and moisten the eyeball. If viruses are rubbed into the eyes, they will get into the nose along with the draining tears. One of the best ways to prevent colds is to keep your hands away from your eyes and nose.

shortened the course of colds. Other researchers said that these excess doses of zinc actually made the immune system function more poorly.

Because colds are caused by hundreds of different viruses, they are difficult to prevent. Flu prevention has made much greater strides.

WHAT TO DO ABOUT THE FLU
Vaccines* are preparations, usually given by shots, that

trigger your body to produce antibodies to a virus. The problem with vaccines is to find an antigen that stimulates antibodies but does not cause an infection. Finding this antigen takes a great deal of ingenious research. Using just one "healthy" or functioning virus might start a serious disease in the person being vaccinated.

This is what happened in the first vaccines known to have been created. In ancient Asia, medical people vaccinated the country folk against smallpox by inoculating them with material taken from the scabs the disease produced on people's skin. Healthy people generally came down with a mild case of the disease. This case left them with antibodies that protected them against serious smallpox outbreaks. The problem was that sometimes the inoculations produced such severe cases of smallpox that people died from the medicine.

In the late 1700s, a British physician, Dr. Edward Jenner, came up with a better solution. He inoculated people against smallpox by removing scabs from cattle suffering from cowpox, a similar though less serious disease. Humans contracted a mild case of cowpox and became immune to episodes of smallpox. Jenner called the infectious agent vaccinia, and the inoculation process vaccination. Both are derived from *vacca*, the Latin word for "cow." This smallpox vaccine is still available today.

Not many human diseases have milder animal counterparts. Scientists have come up with other ways to create unthreatening vaccinations. The flu vaccine you are used to getting makes use of a "killed" or inactivated virus. The vaccine is made by growing a human flu virus in a fertilized egg. The virus is then inactivated with formalin, a formaldehyde solution. (Formaldehyde is the solution in which lab specimens are often preserved.) Formalin sticks to the hemagglutinin and neuraminidase spikes on the surface of the virus, clogging them so they cannot get into human cells. The clogged spikes still trigger an immune response in people, protecting them against infection by this virus.

Because flu viruses change each season, the exact components of the vaccine are different each year. This is why you get vaccinated against the flu once a year, but receive shots against diseases like polio or German measles only once in your lifetime. Every spring, experts from the Food and Drug Administration, the Centers for Disease Control, and other medical groups meet to decide what to put into the next flu season's vaccine. The decision is based on what viruses were circulating the last year, as well as early reports on the flu season in the Southern Hemisphere. The effectiveness of any year's vaccine depends on how well the predicted viruses match the ones that actually spread through the country. When the match is good, about 70 percent of people inoculated and then exposed to the flu do not come down with influenza.

In the 1984–85 season, the vaccine was trivalent. That is, it contained "killed" versions of three flu viruses.

Adults usually get one dose of the flu vaccine, while children under thirteen, who have been exposed to fewer outbreaks, often get two shots. These shots usually produce antibodies in the bloodstream within two weeks. Protection is strong for about six months, then falls off rapidly. The vaccines sometimes cause flulike symptoms, but that does not mean you have become infected. The foreign particle simply has activated some of the immune responses that cause many influenza symptoms.

Scientists are working in at least two directions to make vaccines more effective. One is the making of a giant vaccine. Scientists from the New York State Department of Health have inserted genes from an influenza (or other) virus into the very large vaccinia (cowpox) virus. When animals are inoculated with the vaccinia virus, its influenzalike characteristics fool the immune system into producing antibodies to the flu. Inoculated people run no risk of actually coming down with influenza, because flu viruses themselves are not present. Since vaccinia is an unusually

large virus, several different strains of flu viruses could fit into the vaccine at one time. This would give inoculated people protection from more strains than is currently possible.

A second direction of research is the use of what is known as "live" viruses. Building a "live" virus takes place in two stages. First, scientists breed an influenza virus that thrives only in low temperatures. This means that when it gets into the warmer human body, it will not function. In the second stage, this harmless virus is crossbred with an influenza virus that could cause an infection. A third virus comes out of this mating. This virus has the RNA pieces for the H and N spikes of the infectious flu virus, but its remaining RNA is for the harmless virus. When people are inoculated with the virus, the immune system recognizes the H and N spikes and produces antibodies.

The inoculated virus will not cause an infection because it cannot take over a human cell in the warm environment of the body. In experiments, this "live"-virus vaccine is more effective than the "killed" one. The newer one is delivered by nose drops, producing antibodies in the mucous membranes where they are most needed. So far, these experimental vaccines have only been produced for influenza A viruses, but the prospects of a vaccine against B viruses look good.

If you did not get vaccinated and the flu makes an appearance in your school or neighborhood, there is a fallback option, an antiviral drug known as amantadine. Amantadine is one of about five antiviral medications available to the public. Unlike antibiotics, which do damage to most of the bacteria inside the body, antiviral products are targeted to very specific infectious agents. Amantadine works against the influenza A virus by preventing it from getting completely inside a cell, thus stopping it from reproducing.

Amantadine is 70 to 90 percent effective in preventing infection by influenza A viruses. Doctors prefer using vaccines as preventive measures since amantadine does not work against influenza B. Also, as a way to prevent the flu, amantadine is burdensome. You need to keep taking it for the duration of an epidemic in your area, which generally means six to twelve weeks.

Once you have come down with the flu, amantadine makes the disease last for a shorter period of time, with milder symptoms. A related drug, rimantadine, works as effectively as amantadine and seems to produce fewer side effects. Now used in Russia, the drug is not yet approved for sale in the United States.

Other than taking amantadine, treating the flu is similar to treating a cold. There is one exception. Do not take aspirin if you have the flu. Doctors have found a link between taking aspirin during viral infections such as flu and chicken pox and the onset of a disease called Reye's syndrome. Reye's syndrome is an illness of the liver and brain that kills about one-quarter of its victims, all of whom are children. For the aches and fever of the flu, you are safer taking acetaminophen.

WHAT'S THE FUTURE OF THE COMMON COLD?

Because cold viruses come in so many different forms, each requiring a different antibody, developing a vaccine is not the answer to the common cold. Scientists are looking for other kinds of solutions. Each year a new antiviral drug holds out promise, but the substance with the best track record so far is interferon. The type of interferon used to help prevent colds is the same kind our bodies naturally produce when infected. Up until recently, producing interferon for medicinal purposes was exorbitantly expensive. Interferon is species-specific. That is, only human interferon will work with humans. Interferon from, for instance, a cow, has no effect on human colds. Consequently, interferon could only be made from human blood. In the last few years, however, advances in gene-splicing techniques have allowed manufacturers to mass-produce the substance.

Gene splicing is the process of altering the genetic structure of cells in the laboratory. This newer technique involves putting DNA from an interferon cell into a bacteria cell. The DNA instructs the bacteria to produce not a new bacteria, but a new interferon cell. Interferon works well in stopping colds (it is not as effective in stopping influenza), but it has one drawback. After about seven days of use, the substance starts doing more harm than good. It makes your nose bleed and causes tears in the mucous membranes. Most likely the best use for interferon in the future will be to prevent family members from catching a cold that one person in the family has picked up.

Two other ways to prevent the spread of colds are also being looked into. One is a facial tissue treated with a chemical that kills viruses. When people sneeze or cough into the tissue, known as a Killer Kleenex, they are much less likely than others to pass along their colds. The tissue is made by the Kimberly-Clark Corporation in Neenah, Wisconsin. A less developed approach is to manufacture hand lotion that has a virus-killing chemical inside it. Since colds spread more by hand contact than by sneezing or coughing, this may prove an effective way to stop transmission. With refinement of these techniques and some not even thought up yet, someday the common cold may become an uncommon occurrence.

GLOSSARY

Agglutinate *(ag-GLU-te-nate).* To clump together.

Alveoli *(al-VAY-a-lee).* Air sacs in the lungs.

Antibodies *(AN-ti-BAHD-eez).* Special proteins produced by the immune system that kill off or otherwise disarm invaders.

Anticholinergic *(AN-ti-ko-le-NER-jik).* A class of drug that reduces the flow of fluids in the eyes and nose.

Antigen *(AN-ti-jen).* An intruder that causes the body to produce antibodies.

Antihistamine *(AN-ti-HIS-ta-men).* A type of drug that relieves cold, flu, and allergy symptoms by preventing the release of an internal chemical called histamine.

Antitussive *(AN-ti-TUS-iv).* A type of medicine that signals the brain to stop the coughing reaction.

Bacteria *(back-TEER-ee-a).* Microscopic, one-celled organisms shaped like rods, balls, or spirals. Poisons produced by these organisms when they are inside a body create illness.

Bronchi *(BRON-kee)*. The two large air tubes that enter the right and left lungs.

Bronchioles *(BRON-kee-ols)*. Tiny, thin-walled air tubes that branch out from the bronchi in the lungs.

Cartilage *(KAR-til-ij)*. Tissue that helps hold up the body, but is softer and more flexible than bones.

Enzyme *(EN-zime)*. A class of proteins inside the body that spark chemical reactions.

Epiglottis *(ep-e-GLOT-is)*. A thin piece of cartilage behind the tongue that closes during swallowing to prevent food from going down the windpipe.

Esophagus *(ee-SA-fa-gus)*. The tube through which food passes down from the throat to the stomach.

Expectorant. A type of cough medicine that thins and loosens mucus stuck in the throat and chest.

Hemagglutinin (H) *(HEE-ma-GLOOT-e-nin)*. Protein spikes on the outside of a virus that attach to very specific cells, clearing the way for the virus to take over the cell.

Inflammation *(IN-fla-MAY-shun)*. Soreness, swelling, warmth, and redness that occur when red and white blood cells rush to the scene of an infection.

Interferon *(in-ter-FEER-on)*. A substance produced by the body that makes cells less likely to be taken over by viruses.

Larynx *(LAR-inks)*. The part of the windpipe that contains the vocal cords.

Lower respiratory tract. The lungs and the bronchi.

Lymphatic system *(lim-FA-tik SIS-tem)*. A network of tubes that carries away refuse from cells, plus a set of glands that produce a type of white blood cell.

Lymphocyte *(LIM-fo-site)*. A group of white blood cells that make antibodies, devour bacteria, and otherwise fight off infections.

Macrophage *(MAK-ro-fage)*. "Big eater" white blood cells that consume bacteria and dead cells.

Mucous membranes *(MYOO-kus MEM-branes)*. Tissues in the upper respiratory tract that produce mucus.

58

Mucus *(MYOO-kus).* A thick, slimy substance that moistens and protects passages in the nose, head, and upper throat.

Neuraminidase (N) *(nyoor-a-MIN-ee-days).* A type of spike on the outside of a virus that helps the virus enter a cell.

Pharynx *(FAR-inks).* The upper part of the throat, before the throat splits into the esophagus and windpipe.

Upper respiratory tract. The nasal and oral cavities, sinuses, pharynx, larynx, and trachea.

Vaccine *(vak-SEEN).* A preparation containing germs (usually weakened) introduced into the body to produce immunity, often by means of a shot.

Virus *(VIE-rus).* A class of submicroscopic infectious agents that are not able to reproduce or carry out other living activities until they invade a living cell.

INDEX

ABOUT
THE AUTHOR

Nancy Stedman is a New York-based freelance writer who specializes in health topics. She is a contributing editor to *Health* magazine. Her work has appeared in *Self*, *Ladies Home Journal*, the *New York Times*, the *Christian Science Monitor*, and other publications. Ms. Stedman received a B.A. from the University of Connecticut, and an M.S. from the University of Wisconsin.